CSID DIET COOKBOOK

A Complete Guide to Eating Well with Congenital Sucrase-Isomaltase Deficiency

LILLIAN ROSEWOOD

Table of Contents

INTRODUCTION TO CONGENITAL SUCRASE-ISOMALTASE DEFICIENCY (CSID)

I'm glad you purchase this book to know about your CSID. I know this can be a challenging condition to manage, but I'm here to help you learn more about it and develop a plan to cope with it.

CSID stands for congenital sucrase-isomaltase deficiency. It's a rare genetic disorder that affects the ability to digest sucrose and maltose, two types of sugars. People with CSID have a deficiency of the enzymes sucrase and isomaltase, which are responsible for breaking down these sugars.

The cause of CSID is a genetic mutation that prevents the body from producing enough of the sucrase and isomaltase enzymes. This mutation is inherited in an autosomal recessive manner, which means that both parents must carry the gene for CSID in order for their child to be affected.

In your case, it's likely that you inherited the gene for CSID from one or both of your parents. However, it's also possible that the mutation occurred spontaneously in your genes.

The symptoms of CSID typically begin in early childhood after the introduction of solid foods. Common symptoms include:

- Diarrhea
- Abdominal pain
- Bloating
- Gas
- Weight loss
- Failure to thrive

In some cases, people with CSID may also experience vomiting, nausea, and constipation.

If you're experiencing any of these symptoms, it's important to see a doctor to get a diagnosis. There is no cure for

CSID, but the symptoms can be managed with a special diet and enzyme replacement therapy.

The most important thing you can do to manage your CSID is to avoid foods that contain sucrose and maltose. This includes table sugar, honey, fruit juices, candy, bread, pasta, and cereal.

There are also a number of enzyme replacement therapies that can be used to help you digest sugars. These therapies are typically prescribed by a doctor and can be taken as tablets or capsules.

With proper management, people with CSID can live a normal and healthy life. However, it's important to be aware of the symptoms of the condition and to seek medical attention if they occur.

I know this can be a lot to take in, but I'm here to help you every step of the way.

Importance of Diet in Managing CSID

CSID stands for congenital sucrase-isomaltase deficiency. It's a rare genetic disorder that affects the ability to digest sucrose and maltose, two types of sugars. People with

CSID have a deficiency of the enzymes sucrase and isomaltase, which are responsible for breaking down these sugars.

The most important thing you can do to manage your CSID is to follow a special diet. This diet will help you avoid foods that contain sucrose and maltose, which can cause symptoms like diarrhea, abdominal pain, bloating, gas, and weight loss.

Foods you should avoid if you have CSID:

- Table sugar
- Honey
- Fruit juices
- Candy
- Bread
- Pasta
- Cereal

Foods that are safe for people with CSID

There are also a number of foods that are safe for people with CSID to eat. These foods include:

- Vegetables

- Fruits (without added sugar)

- Lean protein

- Whole grains

- Dairy products (if tolerated)

It's also important to make sure you're getting enough fluids if you have CSID. This will help to prevent dehydration, which can be a complication of the condition.

The Science behind CSID

CSID Diet: Understanding Sucrase and Isomaltase Enzymes

Congenital Sucrase-Isomaltase Deficiency (CSID) is a condition that affects how your body digests certain carbohydrates. To understand CSID, let's break down the role of two important enzymes: sucrase and isomaltase.

Sucrase Enzyme:

Sucrase is an enzyme that your body produces to help break down a sugar called sucrose. Sucrose is commonly found in table sugar and in many foods that have added sugars. When you consume sucrose-containing foods, your body needs sucrase to break down sucrose into simpler sugars like glucose and fructose. These simpler sugars can then be absorbed into your bloodstream and used for energy.

Isomaltase Enzyme:

Isomaltase is another enzyme that plays a crucial role in digestion. It helps break down a type of carbohydrate called isomaltose. Isomaltose is found in starchy foods like grains and potatoes. Similar to sucrase, isomaltase breaks down isomaltose into smaller sugars that your body can absorb and use for energy.

CSID and Enzyme Deficiency:

In people with CSID, there is a deficiency of sucrase and/or isomaltase enzymes. This deficiency means that your body has trouble breaking down sucrose and isomaltose into their simpler forms. As a result, undigested sugars can pass through your digestive system without being properly absorbed. This can lead to uncomfortable symptoms like stomach pain, bloating, gas, and diarrhea after consuming foods that contain sucrose or isomaltose.

Managing CSID with Diet:

Managing CSID involves following a special diet that avoids or limits foods high in sucrose and isomaltose. By choosing foods that are easier for your body to digest, you can reduce the symptoms associated with CSID. Your diet may include options like fruits with lower sugar content, non-starchy vegetables, lean proteins, and certain grains that are better tolerated.

How CSID Impacts Digestion and Nutrient Absorption

Congenital Sucrase-Isomaltase Deficiency (CSID) can have a significant impact on the way your body digests food and absorbs nutrients. To understand how CSID affects digestion and nutrient absorption, let's delve into the process step by step.

Normal Digestion Process:

When you eat, your body starts breaking down the food in your stomach and intestines. Enzymes, like sucrase and isomaltase, play a key role in this process. These enzymes break down complex carbohydrates into simpler sugars that your body can absorb. Once these sugars are broken down, they can enter your bloodstream and provide energy to your cells.

Effects of CSID on Digestion:

In individuals with CSID, there is a deficiency or absence of sucrase and/or isomaltase enzymes. This deficiency makes it difficult for your body to break down certain sugars, such as sucrose and isomaltose, into their basic forms. As a result, these undigested sugars can remain in your digestive system, leading to various symptoms like bloating, gas, stomach discomfort, and diarrhea.

Impact on Nutrient Absorption:

The inability to properly break down sugars due to CSID can affect nutrient absorption in several ways:

1. **Reduced Sugar Absorption:** With a lack of sucrase and isomaltase enzymes, sugars like sucrose and isomaltose cannot be broken down into smaller, absorbable forms. This means that these sugars cannot be efficiently absorbed into your bloodstream.

2. **Limited Nutrient Availability:** Since undigested sugars cannot be absorbed, they may provide a breeding ground for bacteria in the intestines. This bacterial activity can lead to the production of gas and other byproducts, causing discomfort.

3. **Malabsorption of Nutrients:** CSID-related symptoms can also interfere with the absorption of other nutrients, such as vitamins and minerals. This can potentially lead to nutritional deficiencies if not properly managed.

Managing Digestion and Nutrient Absorption with Diet:

To manage CSID and its effects on digestion and nutrient absorption, a carefully planned diet is essential. This diet typically involves avoiding foods high in sucrose and isomaltose, as these are the sugars that your body struggles to break down. Instead, focus on consuming foods that are easier for your body to digest and absorb.

DESIGNING AN EFFECTIVE CSID DIET PLAN

Designing a well-balanced diet plan for individuals with Congenital Sucrase-Isomaltase Deficiency (CSID) requires a thorough understanding of their unique nutritional requirements and the foods that should be avoided. In this chapter, we will delve into the key considerations for creating an effective CSID diet plan.

Nutritional Requirements for CSID Patients:

CSID patients face challenges in digesting and absorbing certain sugars, particularly sucrose and isomaltose. Therefore, crafting a diet that supports their nutritional needs while minimizing discomfort is paramount. Here are the essential components of a CSID diet plan:

1. **Balanced Macronutrients:** Ensure an appropriate balance of carbohydrates, proteins, and fats to meet energy needs. While sugars high in sucrose and isomaltose are

restricted, focus on incorporating complex carbohydrates from sources that are well-tolerated, such as non-starchy vegetables, whole grains, and legumes.

2. **Fiber-Rich Foods:** Include fiber-rich foods to promote healthy digestion. Soluble fiber can help regulate bowel movements and minimize digestive distress. Foods like oats, berries, and beans can be excellent choices.

3. **Lean Proteins:** Opt for lean protein sources like poultry, fish, tofu, and legumes to support muscle health and provide essential amino acids without exacerbating digestive symptoms.

4. **Healthy Fats:** Incorporate sources of healthy fats such as avocados, nuts, seeds, and olive oil. These fats are crucial for overall health and can contribute to satiety.

5. **Vitamins and Minerals:** Ensure an adequate intake of vitamins and minerals by including a variety of nutrient-dense foods. Consider working with a dietitian to monitor potential deficiencies and address them through dietary choices or supplements if necessary.

Foods to Avoid: High Sucrose and Isomaltose Sources:

To prevent digestive discomfort and manage CSID effectively, it's essential to avoid or limit foods that are high in sucrose and isomaltose. These sugars are challenging for individuals with CSID to digest. Here are some examples of foods to avoid or consume in moderation:

1. Table Sugar: Sucrose is a common component of table sugar. Minimize the use of regular sugar in cooking and baking.

2. Processed Foods: Many processed foods contain added sugars, including sucrose and isomaltose. Avoid sugary snacks, candies, and desserts.

3. Sweetened Beverages: Sugary drinks like sodas, fruit juices, and sweetened teas are typically high in sucrose. Opt for water, herbal teas, or beverages sweetened with alternatives like stevia.

4. High-Sugar Fruits: While fruits are generally nutritious, some are higher in sucrose. Limit your intake of fruits like bananas, grapes, and mangoes, and focus on berries, citrus fruits, and melons.

5. Certain Starchy Foods: Some starchy foods like white bread, cakes, and pastries can be high in sucrose and isomaltose. Choose whole-grain alternatives and be mindful of portion sizes.

Creating a CSID diet plan that balances nutritional requirements and restrictions can be intricate.

In the journey of crafting a balanced diet plan for individuals with Congenital Sucrase-Isomaltase Deficiency (CSID), the selection of carbohydrates plays a pivotal role. This chapter delves into the nuances of choosing the right carbohydrates—ones that are low in both sugar and isomaltose content—to support digestive comfort and overall health.

Choosing the Right Carbohydrates: Low-Sugar and Low-Isomaltose Options

When tailoring a diet plan for CSID patients, the focus shifts towards carbohydrates that are well-tolerated and gentle on the digestive system. Here's an exploration of the types of carbohydrates that are optimal for CSID management:

1. Complex Carbohydrates: Opt for carbohydrates that are complex in structure, such as whole grains, legumes, and vegetables. These carbohydrates contain fiber and starches that are broken down more slowly, minimizing the sudden release of sugars that can trigger digestive discomfort.

2. Non-Starchy Vegetables: Vegetables like leafy greens, broccoli, cauliflower, and bell peppers are low in sugars and isomaltose. They offer essential nutrients, vitamins, and minerals without straining the digestive process.

3. Low-Sugar Fruits: Certain fruits are naturally lower in sugar content and can be included in moderation. Berries, melons, and citrus fruits are excellent choices due to their reduced sugar load.

4. Whole Grains: Opt for whole grains like quinoa, brown rice, and oats. These grains contain fiber, which aids digestion and slows the absorption of sugars into the bloodstream.

5. Legumes and Beans: Legumes such as lentils, chickpeas, and black beans are rich in protein, fiber, and complex carbohydrates, making them valuable additions to a CSID diet.

6. Alternative Flours: Explore flours made from alternative sources like almond, coconut, or cassava. These flours can be used in baking and cooking to create CSID-friendly versions of your favorite dishes.

Reading Labels and *Ingredients:*

When selecting packaged foods, reading labels becomes crucial for individuals with CSID. Look for products labeled as "sugar-free," "no added sugars," or "low sugar." Be cautious of hidden sugars or sugar substitutes that might still trigger discomfort.

Portion Control and Individual Tolerance:

Well-tolerated, it's essential to listen to your body's responses. Start with small portions of new foods and observe how your body reacts to them.

Consultation with a Dietitian:

Collaborating with a registered dietitian experienced in CSID management can provide invaluable guidance. They can help identify the best carbohydrate choices based on individual preferences, medical history, and nutritional needs. A dietitian can also assist in creating balanced meal plans that align with the specific dietary requirements of CSID.

In essence, selecting the right carbohydrates for CSID patients involves focusing on complex, low-sugar, and low-isomaltose options. By incorporating these carbohydrate sources into the diet, individuals can nourish their bodies while maintaining digestive comfort and overall well-being.

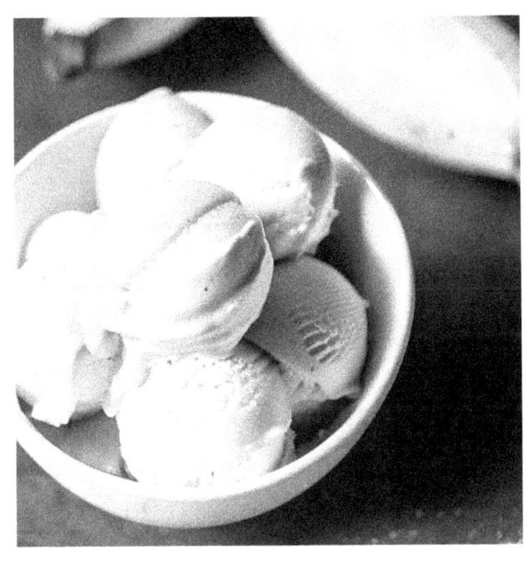

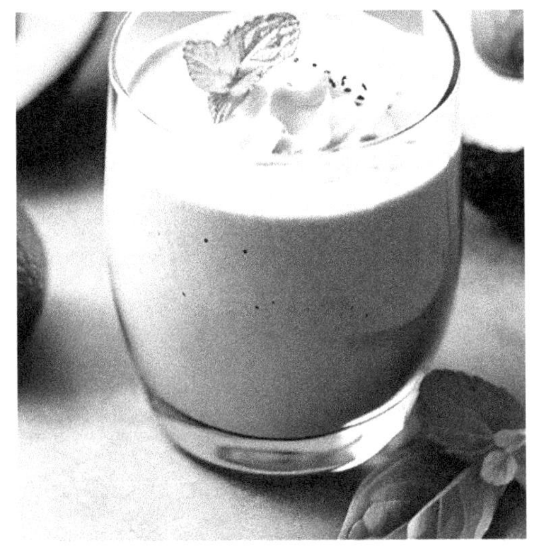

Building a Balanced CSID Meal

A 4 week meal plan

WEEK 1

Day	Breakfast	Lunch	Dinner	Snacks
1	Oatmeal with berries and nuts	Salad with grilled chicken or fish, vegetables, and a vinaigrette dressing	Salmon with roasted vegetables	Fruits and vegetables
2	Eggs with whole-wheat toast and avocado	Soup made with broth, vegetables, and lean protein	Chicken stir-fry with brown rice	Hard-boiled eggs
3	Yogurt with	Sandwich on	Lentil soup	Nuts and

				seeds
	fruit and granola	whole-wheat bread with lean protein, vegetables, and a mustard or vinegar-based spread		
4	Smoothie made with protein powder, milk, fruit, and vegetables	Veggie burger on a whole-wheat bun with toppings of your choice	Tofu scramble with vegetables	Trail mix
5	Pancakes made with buckwheat flour and topped with fruit	Leftovers from dinner	Vegetarian chili	Fruits and vegetables
6	Quinoa Breakfast	Grilled Chicken	Baked Salmon	Apple Slices with

	Bowl:	Salad:	with Roasted Vegetables	Nut Butter
7	Greek Yogurt Parfait	Quinoa Salad with Veggies and Chicken	Stir-Fried Tofu and Vegetable Medley	Carrot Sticks with Hummus

Day 1:

- Breakfast - Oatmeal with Berries and Nuts:

Ingredients:

- 1/2 cup oats

- 1 cup water or lactose-free milk

- 1/4 cup low-sugar berries (blueberries, raspberries)

- 1 tablespoon chopped nuts (almonds, walnuts)

Instructions:

1. In a pot, bring water or lactose-free milk to a boil.

2. Add oats and cook according to package instructions.

3. Top with berries and chopped nuts before serving.

- *Nutrition Information (approximate):*

  - Calories: 250

  - Protein: 8g

  - Carbohydrates: 38g

  - Fat: 8g

  - Fiber: 6g

Lunch - Grilled Chicken or Fish Salad:

- *Ingredients:*

  - 4 oz grilled chicken or fish (salmon)

  - Mixed greens

  - Assorted vegetables (tomatoes, cucumber, bell peppers)

  - Homemade vinaigrette dressing (olive oil, vinegar, herbs)

- *Instructions:*

1. Grill chicken or fish seasoned with herbs.

2. Prepare a salad with mixed greens and assorted vegetables.

3. Top with grilled chicken or fish and drizzle with vinaigrette dressing.

Nutrition Information (approximate):

- Calories: 300-350 (varies based on protein choice)

- Protein: 25-30g

- Carbohydrates: 10-15g

- Fat: 15-20g

- Fiber: 3-5g

Dinner - Baked Salmon with Roasted Vegetables:

- Ingredients:

- 4 oz salmon fillet

- Assorted vegetables (broccoli, carrots, zucchini)

- Olive oil

- Herbs and seasonings

Instructions:

1. Preheat the oven to 375°F (190°C).

2. Place salmon on a baking sheet, brush with olive oil, and season with herbs and spices.

3. Toss chopped vegetables with olive oil, herbs, and seasonings.

4. Bake salmon and vegetables in the oven until cooked through.

Nutrition Information (approximate):

- Calories: 350-400 (varies based on portion sizes)

- Protein: 25-30g

- Carbohydrates: 15-20g

- Fat: 20-25g

- Fiber: 5-7g

Snacks - Fruits and Vegetables:

Ingredients:

- Assorted sliced fruits (apple, pear)

- Assorted cut vegetables (cucumber, bell pepper)

Instructions:

1. Slice fruits and cut vegetables into bite-sized pieces.

2. Enjoy them as refreshing snacks throughout the day.

- Nutrition Information (approximate):

- Varies based on portion sizes and types of fruits/vegetables.

Day 2:

Breakfast - Avocado Toast with Eggs:

- Ingredients:

- 2 eggs

- 2 slices whole-wheat toast

- 1 ripe avocado

- Salt and pepper

Instructions:

1. Toast the whole-wheat bread slices.

2. While the bread is toasting, prepare scrambled or boiled eggs according to your preference.

3. Mash the ripe avocado and spread it onto the toasted bread.

4. Top with the cooked eggs and season with salt and pepper.

Nutrition Information (approximate):

- Calories: 350-400

- Protein: 15-20g

- Carbohydrates: 25-30g

- Fat: 20-25g

- Fiber: 8-10g

Lunch - Vegetable and Lean Protein Soup:

- Ingredients:

  - 4 cups broth (chicken or vegetable)

  - Assorted vegetables (carrots, celery, zucchini)

  - Lean protein (chicken, turkey, beans)

  - Herbs and seasonings

Instructions:

  1. Heat the broth in a pot.

  2. Add chopped vegetables and lean protein to the broth.

  3. Simmer until the vegetables are tender and the protein is cooked through.

  4. Season with herbs and spices to taste.

Nutrition Information (approximate):

  - Calories: 250-300

  - Protein: 15-20g

  - Carbohydrates: 20-25g

- Fat: 10-15g

- Fiber: 5-7g

Dinner - Chicken Stir-Fry with Brown Rice:

Ingredients:

- 4 oz lean chicken breast, sliced

- Assorted vegetables (broccoli, bell peppers, snap peas)

- Low-sodium soy sauce

- Cooked brown rice

Instructions:

1. In a pan, stir-fry sliced chicken until cooked.

2. Add chopped vegetables and stir-fry until tender-crisp.

3. Season with a drizzle of low-sodium soy sauce.

4. Serve over cooked brown rice.

Nutrition Information (approximate):

- Calories: 350-400

- Protein: 25-30g

- Carbohydrates: 30-35g

- Fat: 10-15g

- Fiber: 5-7g

Snacks - Hard-Boiled Eggs:

Ingredients:

- Eggs

Instructions:

1. Hard-boil eggs by placing them in boiling water for about 10-12 minutes.

2. Peel and enjoy as a convenient protein-rich snack.

Nutrition Information (approximate):

- Calories: 70-80

- Protein: 6g

- Carbohydrates: 1g

- Fat: 5g

- Fiber: 0g

Day 3:

Breakfast - Fruit and Yogurt Parfait:

Ingredients:

- 1 cup lactose-free Greek yogurt

- 1/2 cup mixed low-sugar fruits (berries, kiwi)

- 2 tablespoons granola

Instructions:

1. In a glass or bowl, layer Greek yogurt, mixed fruits, and granola.

2. Repeat the layers as desired.

Nutrition Information (approximate):

- Calories: 250-300

- Protein: 15-20g

- Carbohydrates: 35-40g

- Fat: 8-10g

- Fiber: 5-7g

Lunch - Lean Protein Sandwich:

Ingredients:

- Lean protein (turkey, chicken)

- Whole-wheat bread

- Assorted vegetables (lettuce, tomato, cucumber)

- Mustard or vinegar-based spread

Instructions:

1. Assemble a sandwich with lean protein, whole-wheat bread, and vegetables.

2. Spread mustard or a vinegar-based dressing for flavor.

Nutrition Information (approximate):

- Calories: 300-350

- Protein: 20-25g

- Carbohydrates: 30-35g

- Fat: 10-12g

- Fiber: 5-7g

Dinner - Hearty Lentil Soup:

Ingredients:

- 1 cup lentils

- Assorted vegetables (carrots, celery, onion)

- Vegetable or chicken broth

- Herbs and spices

Instructions:

1. Rinse lentils and cook according to package instructions.

2. In a pot, sauté chopped vegetables until tender.

3. Add cooked lentils and enough broth to cover the ingredients.

4. Simmer until flavors are well combined.

Nutrition Information (approximate):

- Calories: 300-350

- Protein: 15-20g

- Carbohydrates: 50-55g

- Fat: 5-7g

- Fiber: 15-20g

Snacks - Nuts and Seeds:

Ingredients:

- Mixed nuts (almonds, walnuts, cashews)

- Mixed seeds (sunflower seeds, pumpkin seeds)

Instructions:

1. Create a custom mix of nuts and seeds for a satisfying snack.

Nutrition Information (approximate):

- Varies based on portion sizes and types of nuts/seeds.

Day 4:

Breakfast - Protein-Packed Smoothie:

Ingredients:

- 1 scoop protein powder (lactose-free)

- 1 cup lactose-free milk

- 1/2 cup mixed low-sugar fruits (berries, banana)

- Handful of spinach or kale

- 1 tablespoon nut butter

Instructions:

1. Blend protein powder, lactose-free milk, fruits, greens, and nut butter until smooth.

Nutrition Information (approximate):

- Calories: 350-400

- Protein: 25-30g

- Carbohydrates: 30-35g

- Fat: 15-20g

- Fiber: 5-7g

Lunch - Veggie Burger on a Bun:

Ingredients:

- 1 veggie burger patty

- 1 whole-wheat bun

- Assorted toppings (lettuce, tomato, onion)

- Condiments of choice (mustard, ketchup)

Instructions:

1. Cook the veggie burger patty according to package instructions.

2. Assemble the burger with whole-wheat bun, veggie patty, and assorted toppings.

Nutrition Information (approximate):

- Calories: 300-350

- Protein: 15-20g

- Carbohydrates: 40-45g

- Fat: 10-15g

- Fiber: 8-10g

Dinner - Tofu and Vegetable Stir-Fry:

Ingredients:

- 6 oz firm tofu, cubed

- Assorted vegetables (broccoli, bell peppers, carrots)

- Low-sodium soy sauce

- Olive oil

Instructions:

1. Sauté cubed tofu in a pan with a small amount of olive oil until lightly browned.

2. Add chopped vegetables and stir-fry until tender.

3. Season with low-sodium soy sauce.

Nutrition Information (approximate):

- Calories: 300-350

- Protein: 20-25g

- Carbohydrates: 25-30g

- Fat: 12-15g

- Fiber: 5-7g

Snacks - Trail Mix:

Ingredients:

- Mixed nuts (almonds, cashews)

- Dried fruits (raisins, cranberries)

- Seeds (pumpkin seeds, sunflower seeds)

Instructions:

1. Create a customized trail mix using a variety of nuts, dried fruits, and seeds.

Nutrition Information (approximate):

- Varies based on portion sizes and types of ingredients.

Day 5:

Breakfast - Buckwheat Pancakes with Fruit:

Ingredients:

- 1/2 cup buckwheat flour

- 1/2 teaspoon baking powder

- 1 egg

- 1/2 cup lactose-free milk

- 1/2 teaspoon vanilla extract

- Mixed low-sugar fruits (berries, sliced banana)

Instructions:

1. In a bowl, whisk together buckwheat flour and baking powder.

2. In a separate bowl, beat the egg, then add lactose-free milk and vanilla extract.

3. Combine wet and dry ingredients until just mixed.

4. Heat a non-stick skillet over medium heat and ladle the batter to make pancakes.

5. Cook until bubbles form on the surface, then flip and cook until golden.

Nutrition Information (approximate):

- Calories: 250-300

- Protein: 8-10g

- Carbohydrates: 40-45g

- Fat: 5-7g

- Fiber: 5-7g

Lunch - Leftovers from Dinner:

 - Instructions:

- Enjoy any remaining dinner from a previous night as a convenient lunch option.

Dinner - Vegetarian Chili:

Ingredients:

- 1 cup mixed beans (kidney beans, black beans)

- Assorted vegetables (bell peppers, onion, zucchini)

- 1 can diced tomatoes

- Low-sodium vegetable broth

- Chili powder, cumin, and other spices

Instructions:

1. Sauté chopped vegetables in a pot until tender.

2. Add mixed beans, diced tomatoes, and enough vegetable broth to cover the ingredients.

3. Season with chili powder, cumin, and other desired spices.

4. Simmer until flavors meld together.

Nutrition Information (approximate):

- Calories: 300-350

- Protein: 15-20g

- Carbohydrates: 50-55g

- Fat: 5-7g

- Fiber: 15-20g

Snacks - Fruits and Vegetables:

- Ingredients:

- Assorted sliced fruits (apple, pear)

- Assorted cut vegetables (cucumber, bell pepper)

Instructions:

- Snack on sliced fruits and vegetables throughout the day for a light and refreshing treat.

Nutrition Information (approximate):

- Varies based on portion sizes and types of fruits/vegetables.

Day 6:

Breakfast - Quinoa Breakfast Bowl:

- Ingredients:

  - 1/2 cup cooked quinoa

  - 1/4 cup diced strawberries

  - 1 small banana, sliced

  - 1 tablespoon almond butter (if tolerated)

  - Cinnamon for flavor

- Instructions:

1. Cook quinoa according to package instructions.

2.   In a bowl, combine cooked quinoa, diced strawberries, banana slices, and almond butter.

3.   Sprinkle with cinnamon for extra flavor.

Nutritional Information (approximate):

- Calories: ~300 kcal

- Carbohydrates: ~45g

- Protein: ~6g

- Fat: ~10g

- Fiber: ~6g

Lunch - Grilled Chicken Salad:

- Ingredients:

  - 4 oz grilled chicken breast, sliced

  - Mixed salad greens (e.g., lettuce, spinach)

  - 1/4 cup cucumber slices

  - 1/4 cup cherry tomatoes, halved

  - Olive oil and lemon juice for dressing

- Instructions:

1. Arrange the mixed salad greens on a plate.

2. Top with grilled chicken slices, cucumber, and cherry tomatoes.

3. Drizzle with a small amount of olive oil and lemon juice for dressing.

Nutritional Information (approximate):

- Calories: ~250 kcal

- Carbohydrates: ~8g

- Protein: ~30g

- Fat: ~10g

- Fiber: ~3g

Snack - Apple Slices with Nut Butter:

- Ingredients:

- 1 medium apple, sliced

- 1 tablespoon almond butter (if tolerated)

- Instructions:

1. Wash and slice the apple.

2. Dip the apple slices into almond butter for a satisfying snack.

   Nutritional Information (approximate):

   - Calories: ~150 kcal

   - Carbohydrates: ~25g

   - Protein: ~2g

   - Fat: ~6g

   - Fiber: ~5g

Dinner - Baked Salmon with Roasted Vegetables:

- Ingredients:

  - 6 oz salmon fillet

  - Assorted vegetables (e.g., zucchini, bell peppers, carrots), cut into chunks

  - Olive oil for drizzling

- Lemon juice for flavor

- Fresh herbs (e.g., dill, thyme), chopped

- Salt and pepper to taste

- Instructions:

1. Preheat the oven to 375°F (190°C).

2. Place salmon fillet on a baking sheet. Drizzle with olive oil and lemon juice.

3. Season with chopped herbs, salt, and pepper.

4. On a separate baking sheet, spread the chopped vegetables. Drizzle with olive oil, salt, and pepper.

5. Bake both the salmon and vegetables for about 15-20 minutes or until salmon flakes easily and vegetables are tender.

Nutritional Information (approximate):

- Calories: ~400 kcal

- Carbohydrates: ~10g

- Protein: ~30g

- Fat: ~25g

- Fiber: ~4g

Day 7:

Breakfast - Greek Yogurt Parfait:

- Ingredients:

    - 1 cup plain Greek yogurt (lactose-free, if needed)

    - 1/4 cup blueberries

    - 1/4 cup diced pineapple (if tolerated)

    - 1 tablespoon chopped nuts (e.g., almonds, walnuts)

- Instructions:

1. In a glass or bowl, layer Greek yogurt, blueberries, diced pineapple, and chopped nuts.

2. Repeat layers as desired.

    Nutritional Information (approximate):

- Calories: ~300 kcal

- Carbohydrates: ~25g

- Protein: ~18g

- Fat: ~15g

- Fiber: ~4g

Lunch - Quinoa Salad with Veggies and Chicken:

- Ingredients:

  - 1/2 cup cooked quinoa

  - 4 oz cooked chicken breast, diced

  - Mixed vegetables (e.g., bell peppers, cherry tomatoes, cucumber), diced

  - Lemon vinaigrette (lemon juice, olive oil, herbs)

- Instructions:

1. In a bowl, combine cooked quinoa, diced chicken, and mixed vegetables.

2. Drizzle with lemon vinaigrette and toss to combine.

Nutritional Information (approximate):

- Calories: ~350 kcal

- Carbohydrates: ~30g

- Protein: ~30g

- Fat: ~12g

- Fiber: ~5g

Snack - Carrot Sticks with Hummus:

- Ingredients:

  - Carrot sticks

  - Hummus

- Instructions:

1. Wash and cut carrot sticks.

2. Serve with hummus for a crunchy and satisfying snack.

Nutritional Information (approximate):

- Calories: ~150 kcal

- Carbohydrates: ~15g

- Protein: ~4g

- Fat: ~8g

- Fiber: ~4g

Dinner - Stir-Fried Tofu and Vegetable Medley:

- Ingredients:

  - 6 oz firm tofu, cubed

  - Assorted vegetables (e.g., broccoli, bell peppers, snap peas), sliced

  - Low-sodium soy sauce

  - Minced garlic and ginger

  - Sesame oil for flavor

  - Crushed red pepper flakes (optional)

- Instructions:

1.   Heat a pan or wok over medium-high heat. Add a small amount of sesame oil.

2.   Add minced garlic and ginger, and sauté for a minute.

3.   Add tofu cubes and stir-fry until lightly browned.

4.   Add sliced vegetables and continue stir-frying until vegetables are tender-crisp.

5.   Drizzle with low-sodium soy sauce and a dash of crushed red pepper flakes for extra flavor.

Nutritional Information (approximate):

- Calories: ~300 kcal

- Carbohydrates: ~20g

- Protein: ~20g

- Fat: ~18g

- Fiber: ~6g

Week 2

Day	Breakfast	Lunch	Dinner	Snacks
8	Overnight oats with berries and chia seeds	Salad with chickpeas, vegetables, and a tahini dressing	Salmon with roasted vegetables	Hard-boiled eggs
9	Scrambled eggs with vegetables	Soup made with lentils, vegetables, and a curry dressing	Chicken stir-fry with brown rice	Nuts and seeds
10	Yogurt parfait with granola and berries	Sandwich on whole-wheat bread with lean protein, vegetables, and hummus	Lentil soup	Trail mix
11	Smoothie made with protein	Veggie burger on a whole-wheat	Tofu scramble with	Fruits and vegetables

	powder, milk, fruit, and spinach	bun with toppings of your choice	vegetables	
12	Pancakes made with buckwheat flour and topped with fruit	Leftovers from dinner	Vegetarian chili	Fruits and vegetables
13	Banana Oat Pancakes	Spinach and Chickpea Salad	Turkey and Vegetable Stir-Fry	Rice Cakes with Peanut Butter
14	Scrambled Eggs with Spinach	Lentil and Vegetable Soup	Rice Crackers with Sliced Cheese	Grilled Shrimp with Roasted Asparagus

Day 8:

Breakfast - Overnight Oats with Berries and Chia Seeds:

Ingredients:

- 1/2 cup oats

- 1 cup lactose-free milk

- 1/4 cup low-sugar berries (blueberries, strawberries)

- 1 tablespoon chia seeds

Instructions:

1. In a jar, combine oats, lactose-free milk, and chia seeds.

2. Stir well, then cover and refrigerate overnight.

3. In the morning, top with berries before serving.

Nutrition Information (approximate):

- Calories: 250-300

- Protein: 10-15g

- Carbohydrates: 35-40g

- Fat: 8-10g

- Fiber: 7-9g

Lunch - Chickpea Salad with Tahini Dressing:

- Ingredients:

  - 1 cup mixed greens

  - 1/2 cup chickpeas (canned, drained)

  - Assorted vegetables (cucumber, bell pepper, tomato)

  - Tahini dressing (tahini, lemon juice, garlic)

Instructions:

1. Toss mixed greens, chickpeas, and chopped vegetables in a bowl.

2. Drizzle with tahini dressing and toss to coat.

Nutrition Information (approximate):

  - Calories: 300-350

  - Protein: 10-15g

  - Carbohydrates: 40-45g

  - Fat: 12-15g

  - Fiber: 8-10g

Dinner - Baked Salmon with Roasted Vegetables:

Ingredients:

- 4 oz salmon fillet

- Assorted vegetables (broccoli, carrots, zucchini)

- Olive oil

- Herbs and seasonings

Instructions:

1. Preheat the oven to 375°F (190°C).

2. Place salmon on a baking sheet, brush with olive oil, and season with herbs and spices.

3. Toss chopped vegetables with olive oil, herbs, and seasonings.

4. Bake salmon and vegetables in the oven until cooked through.

Nutrition Information (approximate):

- Calories: 350-400

- Protein: 25-30g

- Carbohydrates: 15-20g

- Fat: 20-25g

- Fiber: 5-7g

Snacks - Hard-Boiled Eggs:

Ingredients:

- Eggs

Instructions:

1. Hard-boil eggs by placing them in boiling water for about 10-12 minutes.

2. Peel and enjoy as a convenient protein-rich snack.

Nutrition Information (approximate):

- Calories: 70-80

- Protein: 6g

- Carbohydrates: 1g

- Fat: 5g

- Fiber: 0g

Day 9:

Breakfast - Scrambled Eggs with Vegetables:

Ingredients:

- 2 eggs

- Assorted vegetables (bell peppers, spinach, onion)

- Olive oil

- Herbs and seasonings

Instructions:

1. In a pan, sauté chopped vegetables in a small amount of olive oil until tender.

2. Beat eggs and pour them over the vegetables.

3. Scramble until cooked through, seasoning with herbs and seasonings.

Nutrition Information (approximate):

- Calories: 250-300

- Protein: 15-20g

- Carbohydrates: 10-15g

- Fat: 15-20g

- Fiber: 5-7g

Lunch - Lentil Vegetable Soup with Curry Dressing:

Ingredients:

- 1 cup cooked lentils

- Assorted vegetables (carrots, celery, onion)

- Low-sodium vegetable broth

- Curry dressing (curry powder, yogurt, lemon juice)

Instructions:

1. Combine cooked lentils and chopped vegetables in a pot with vegetable broth.

2. Simmer until flavors meld together.

3. Prepare curry dressing by mixing curry powder, yogurt, and lemon juice.

4. Drizzle the dressing over the soup before serving.

Nutrition Information (approximate):

- Calories: 250-300

- Protein: 10-15g

- Carbohydrates: 40-45g

- Fat: 5-7g

- Fiber: 15-20g

Dinner - Chicken Stir-Fry with Brown Rice:

Ingredients:

- 4 oz lean chicken breast, sliced

- Assorted vegetables (broccoli, bell peppers, snap peas)

- Low-sodium soy sauce

- Olive oil

- Cooked brown rice

Instructions:

1. In a pan, stir-fry sliced chicken until cooked.

2. Add chopped vegetables and stir-fry until tender.

3. Season with a drizzle of low-sodium soy sauce.

4. Serve over cooked brown rice.

Nutrition Information (approximate):

- Calories: 350-400

- Protein: 25-30g

- Carbohydrates: 30-35g

- Fat: 10-15g

- Fiber: 5-7g

Snacks - Nuts and Seeds:

Ingredients:

- Mixed nuts (almonds, walnuts, cashews)

- Mixed seeds (sunflower seeds, pumpkin seeds)

Instructions:

1. Create a custom mix of nuts and seeds for a satisfying snack.

Nutrition Information (approximate):

- Varies based on portion sizes and types of nuts/seeds.

Day 10:

Breakfast - Yogurt Parfait with Granola and Berries:

Ingredients:

- 1 cup lactose-free yogurt

- 1/4 cup granola

- 1/4 cup low-sugar berries (blueberries, raspberries)

Instructions:

1. In a glass or bowl, layer lactose-free yogurt, granola, and berries.

2. Repeat the layers as desired.

Nutrition Information (approximate):

- Calories: 300-350

- Protein: 15-20g

- Carbohydrates: 40-45g

- Fat: 10-12g

- Fiber: 5-7g

Lunch - Lean Protein Sandwich with Hummus:

Ingredients:

- Lean protein (turkey, chicken)

- Whole-wheat bread

- Assorted vegetables (lettuce, tomato, cucumber)

- Hummus

Instructions:

1. Assemble a sandwich with lean protein, whole-wheat bread, and vegetables.

2. Spread hummus for added flavor and creaminess.

Nutrition Information (approximate):

- Calories: 300-350

- Protein: 20-25g

- Carbohydrates: 30-35g

- Fat: 10-12g

- Fiber: 5-7g

Dinner - Hearty Lentil Soup:

- *Ingredients:*

  - 1 cup lentils

  - Assorted vegetables (carrots, celery, onion)

  - Vegetable or chicken broth

  - Herbs and spices

Instructions:

1. Rinse lentils and cook according to package instructions.

2. In a pot, sauté chopped vegetables until tender.

3. Add cooked lentils and enough broth to cover the ingredients.

4. Simmer until flavors are well combined.

Nutrition Information (approximate):

- Calories: 300-350

- Protein: 15-20g

- Carbohydrates: 50-55g

- Fat: 5-7g

- Fiber: 15-20g

Snacks - Trail Mix:

Ingredients:

- Mixed nuts (almonds, cashews)

- Dried fruits (raisins, cranberries)

- Seeds (pumpkin seeds, sunflower seeds)

Instructions:

1. Create a customized trail mix using a variety of nuts, dried fruits, and seeds.

Nutrition Information (approximate):

- Varies based on portion sizes and types of ingredients.

Day 11:

Breakfast - Green Protein Smoothie:

Ingredients:

- 1 scoop protein powder (lactose-free)

- 1 cup lactose-free milk

- 1/2 cup mixed low-sugar fruits (berries, banana)

- Handful of spinach

Instructions:

1. Blend protein powder, lactose-free milk, fruits, and spinach until smooth.

Nutrition Information (approximate):

- Calories: 300-350

- Protein: 20-25g

- Carbohydrates: 30-35g

- Fat: 10-12g

- Fiber: 5-7g

Lunch - Veggie Burger with Toppings and Hummus:

Ingredients:

- 1 veggie burger patty

- 1 whole-wheat bun

- Assorted toppings (lettuce, tomato, onion)

- Hummus

Instructions:

1. Cook the veggie burger patty according to package instructions.

2. Assemble the burger with whole-wheat bun, veggie patty, and assorted toppings.

3. Spread hummus on the bun for extra flavor.

Nutrition Information (approximate):

- Calories: 300-350

- Protein: 15-20g

- Carbohydrates: 40-45g

- Fat: 10-12g

- Fiber: 8-10g

Dinner - Tofu Scramble with Vegetables:

Ingredients:

- 6 oz firm tofu, crumbled

- Assorted vegetables (bell peppers, spinach, onion)

- Olive oil

- Turmeric, cumin, and other spices

Instructions:

1. In a pan, sauté chopped vegetables in a small amount of olive oil until tender.

2. Add crumbled tofu and cook, seasoning with turmeric, cumin, and other desired spices.

Nutrition Information (approximate):

- Calories: 250-300

- Protein: 15-20g

- Carbohydrates: 10-15g

- Fat: 15-20g

- Fiber: 5-7g

Snacks - Assorted Fruits and Vegetables:

Ingredients:

- Assorted sliced fruits (apple, pear)

- Assorted cut vegetables (cucumber, bell pepper)

Instructions:

- Enjoy sliced fruits and vegetables as a refreshing and nutritious snack.

Nutrition Information (approximate):

- Varies based on portion sizes and types of fruits/vegetables.

Day 12:

Breakfast - Buckwheat Pancakes with Fruit:

Ingredients:

- 1/2 cup buckwheat flour

- 1/2 teaspoon baking powder

- 1 egg

- 1/2 cup lactose-free milk

- 1/2 teaspoon vanilla extract

- Mixed low-sugar fruits (berries, sliced banana)

Instructions:

1. In a bowl, whisk together buckwheat flour and baking powder.

2. In a separate bowl, beat the egg, then add lactose-free milk and vanilla extract.

3. Combine wet and dry ingredients until just mixed.

4. Heat a non-stick skillet over medium heat and ladle the batter to make pancakes.

5. Cook until bubbles form on the surface, then flip and cook until golden.

Nutrition Information (approximate):

- Calories: 250-300

- Protein: 8-10g

- Carbohydrates: 40-45g

- Fat: 5-7g

- Fiber: 5-7g

Lunch - Leftovers from Dinner:

Instructions:

- Enjoy any remaining dinner from a previous night as a convenient lunch option.

Dinner - Vegetarian Chili:

Ingredients:

- 1 cup mixed beans (kidney beans, black beans)

- Assorted vegetables (bell peppers, onion, zucchini)

- 1 can diced tomatoes

- Low-sodium vegetable broth

- Herbs and spices

Instructions:

1. Sauté chopped vegetables in a pot until tender.

2. Add mixed beans, diced tomatoes, and enough vegetable broth to cover the ingredients.

3. Season with chili powder, cumin, and other spices.

4. Simmer until flavors meld together.

Nutrition Information (approximate):

- Calories: 300-350

- Protein: 15-20g

- Carbohydrates: 50-55g

- Fat: 5-7g

- Fiber: 15-20g

Day 13:

Breakfast - Banana Oat Pancakes:

Ingredients:

- 1 ripe banana, mashed

- 1/2 cup oats (gluten-free, if needed)

- 2 eggs

- 1/2 teaspoon vanilla extract

- Cinnamon for flavor

- Coconut oil for cooking

Instructions:

- In a bowl, mix mashed banana, oats, eggs, vanilla extract, and a pinch of cinnamon.
- Heat coconut oil in a pan over medium heat.
- Pour small portions of the batter onto the pan and cook until bubbles form on the surface. Flip and cook until golden brown.

Nutritional Information (approximate):

- Calories: ~350 kcal

- Carbohydrates: ~45g

- Protein: ~12g

- Fat: ~14g

- Fiber: ~5g

Lunch - Spinach and Chickpea Salad:

- Ingredients:

- 2 cups fresh spinach leaves

- 1/2 cup cooked chickpeas

- 1/4 cup diced cucumbers

- 1/4 cup diced red bell pepper

- Olive oil and balsamic vinegar for dressing

Instructions:

- In a bowl, combine spinach, chickpeas, cucumbers, and red bell pepper.
- Drizzle with a small amount of olive oil and balsamic vinegar for dressing.

Nutritional Information (approximate):

- Calories: ~250 kcal

- Carbohydrates: ~30g

- Protein: ~9g

- Fat: ~10g

- Fiber: ~8g

Snack - Rice Cakes with Peanut Butter:

Ingredients:

- Rice cakes

- Peanut butter (if tolerated)

Instructions:

3.   Spread a thin layer of peanut butter on rice cakes for a satisfying and crunchy snack.

Nutritional Information (approximate):

- Calories: ~200 kcal

- Carbohydrates: ~20g

- Protein: ~6g

- Fat: ~10g

- Fiber: ~2g

Dinner - Turkey and Vegetable Stir-Fry:

Ingredients:

- 6 oz ground turkey

- Mixed stir-fry vegetables (e.g., broccoli, carrots, snap peas)

- Low-sodium soy sauce

- Ginger and garlic for flavor

- Sesame oil for cooking

Instructions:

6.   Heat sesame oil in a pan or wok over medium-high heat.

7.   Add ground turkey and cook until browned.

8.   Add mixed vegetables, minced ginger, and garlic. Stir-fry until vegetables are tender.

9.   Drizzle with low-sodium soy sauce for flavor.

Nutritional Information (approximate):

- Calories: ~350 kcal

- Carbohydrates: ~15g

- Protein: ~30g

- Fat: ~20g

- Fiber: ~5g

Day 14:

Breakfast - Scrambled Eggs with Spinach:

Ingredients:

- 2 eggs

- Handful of fresh spinach leaves

- Salt and pepper to taste

- Coconut oil for cooking

Instructions:

- Heat coconut oil in a pan over medium heat.
- Whisk eggs in a bowl and pour into the pan.
- Add fresh spinach leaves and cook, stirring, until eggs are scrambled and spinach is wilted.
- Season with salt and pepper.

Nutritional Information (approximate):

- Calories: ~250 kcal

- Carbohydrates: ~2g

- Protein: ~18g

- Fat: ~18g

- Fiber: ~1g

Lunch - Lentil and Vegetable Soup:

Ingredients:

- 1 cup cooked lentils

- Mixed vegetables (e.g., carrots, celery, zucchini), diced

- Low-sodium vegetable broth

- Herbs and spices for flavor (e.g., thyme, cumin)

- Olive oil for cooking

Instructions:

- In a pot, heat olive oil and sauté mixed vegetables until slightly softened.
- Add cooked lentils and enough low-sodium vegetable broth to cover the ingredients.
- Season with herbs and spices and let the soup simmer until vegetables are tender.

Nutritional Information (approximate):

- Calories: ~300 kcal

- Carbohydrates: ~45g

- Protein: ~15g

- Fat: ~6g

- Fiber: ~15g

Snack - Rice Crackers with Sliced Cheese:

Ingredients:

- Rice crackers

- Sliced lactose-free cheese (if needed)

Instructions:

Top rice crackers with sliced cheese for a simple and satisfying snack.

Nutritional Information (approximate):

- Calories: ~200 kcal

- Carbohydrates: ~20g

- Protein: ~6g

- Fat: ~10g

- Fiber: ~1g

Dinner - Grilled Shrimp with Roasted Asparagus:

Ingredients:

- 6 oz shrimp, peeled and deveined

- Asparagus spears

- Lemon juice and zest

- Olive oil for drizzling

- Fresh herbs (e.g., parsley, thyme) for flavor

- Salt and pepper to taste

Instructions:

- Preheat the grill or grill pan.

- Toss shrimp with olive oil, lemon zest, and chopped herbs. Season with salt and pepper.
- Grill shrimp until opaque and cooked through.
- Drizzle asparagus spears with olive oil and roast in the oven until tender.
- Serve grilled shrimp with roasted asparagus, drizzled with lemon juice.

Nutritional Information (approximate):

- Calories: ~300 kcal
- Carbohydrates: ~10g
- Protein: ~30g
- Fat: ~15g
- Fiber: ~4g

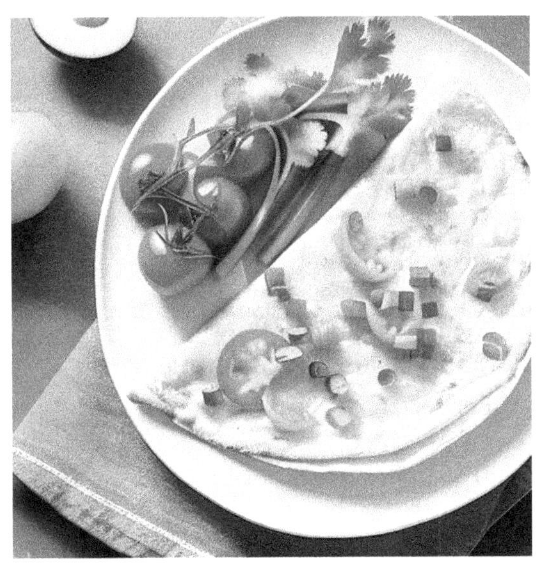

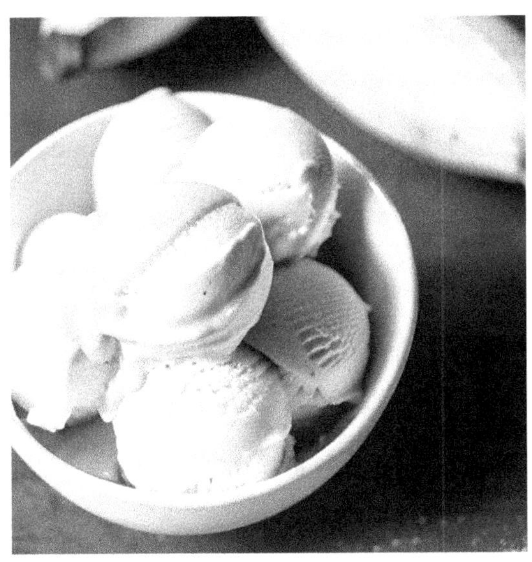

BONUS RECIPES

Smoothies:

1. Berry Delight Smoothie:

- Ingredients: Mixed berries (blueberries, strawberries, raspberries), almond milk (lactose-free), banana (if tolerated), spinach, chia seeds.

- Instructions: Blend all ingredients until smooth.

2. Green Energizer Smoothie:

- Ingredients: Spinach, cucumber, kiwi, pineapple (if tolerated), coconut water.

- Instructions: Blend all ingredients until well combined.

3. Creamy Avocado Smoothie:

- Ingredients: Avocado, banana (if tolerated), almond milk, vanilla extract, a touch of honey (if tolerated).

- Instructions: Blend until creamy and smooth.

4. Tropical Paradise Smoothie:

- Ingredients: Mango (if tolerated), pineapple (if tolerated), coconut milk (lactose-free), lime juice, fresh mint.

- Instructions: Blend until tropical flavors meld.

Breakfast:

5. Omelette with Veggies:

- Ingredients: Eggs, diced bell peppers, diced tomatoes, spinach, olive oil.

- Instructions: Cook veggies in olive oil, pour beaten eggs over, cook until set.

6. Quinoa Breakfast Bowl:

- Ingredients: Cooked quinoa, diced apples, chopped nuts, cinnamon, almond milk.

- Instructions: Mix ingredients in a bowl.

7. Chia Seed Pudding:

- Ingredients: Chia seeds, coconut milk (lactose-free), vanilla extract, fresh berries.

- Instructions: Mix chia seeds, coconut milk, and vanilla. Refrigerate until pudding consistency. Top with berries.

8. Coconut Yogurt Parfait:

- Ingredients: Dairy-free coconut yogurt, granola (CSID-friendly), mixed berries.

- Instructions: Layer yogurt, granola, and berries.

Lunch:

9. Grilled Chicken Salad:

- Ingredients: Grilled chicken strips, mixed greens, cucumber, bell peppers, balsamic vinaigrette.

- Instructions: Assemble ingredients in a bowl.

10. Salmon and Avocado Wrap:

- Ingredients: Grilled salmon, sliced avocado, lettuce leaves, gluten-free wrap (if tolerated).

- Instructions: Layer ingredients in the wrap and roll.

11. Quinoa and Roasted Vegetable Bowl:

- Ingredients: Cooked quinoa, roasted vegetables (zucchini, carrots, bell peppers), olive oil, lemon juice.

- Instructions: Combine ingredients and drizzle with olive oil and lemon juice.

12. Black Bean and Corn Salad:

- Ingredients: Cooked black beans, corn kernels, diced tomatoes, chopped cilantro, lime juice.

- Instructions: Mix all ingredients and season.

Dinner:

13. Grilled Shrimp Skewers:

- Ingredients: Grilled shrimp, bell pepper and onion chunks, olive oil, lemon juice, garlic.

- Instructions: Thread shrimp and veggies onto skewers. Grill until cooked.

14. Stuffed Bell Peppers:

- Ingredients: Bell peppers, ground turkey, diced tomatoes, quinoa, spices.

- Instructions: Hollow peppers, fill with turkey-quinoa mixture, bake.

15. Baked Chicken and Asparagus:

- Ingredients: Baked chicken breast, roasted asparagus, olive oil, lemon zest, herbs.

- Instructions: Season chicken, bake alongside asparagus.

16. Turkey Lettuce Wraps:

- Ingredients: Ground turkey, lettuce leaves, diced water chestnuts, green onions, tamari sauce.

- Instructions: Cook turkey, mix with other ingredients, serve in lettuce wraps.

Desserts:

17. Baked Apples with Cinnamon:

- Ingredients: Apples, cinnamon, chopped nuts (if tolerated).

- Instructions: Core apples, sprinkle with cinnamon and nuts, bake until tender.

18. Banana "Ice Cream":

- Ingredients: Frozen bananas, vanilla extract (if tolerated).

- Instructions: Blend frozen bananas until creamy.

19. Coconut Macaroons:

- Ingredients: Shredded coconut, egg whites, vanilla extract (if tolerated).

- Instructions: Mix ingredients, shape into macaroons, bake until golden.

20. Chocolate Avocado Mousse:

- Ingredients: Avocado, cocoa powder, honey (if tolerated), vanilla extract.

- Instructions: Blend until smooth and creamy.

NAVIGATING RESTAURANTS AND SOCIAL SITUATIONS

Tips for Dining Out with CSID

Here are some tips for navigating restaurants and social situations as a CSID patient:

- Do your research. Before you go to a restaurant, take some time to look at the menu online or call ahead to ask about the ingredients in the dishes. This will help you avoid any surprises when you order.

- Be prepared to ask questions. If you're not sure about an ingredient, don't be afraid to ask the waiter or waitress. They should be happy to help you find something that you can eat.

- Order safe foods. If you're not sure what to order, there are a few safe foods that you can always count on. These include grilled meats and vegetables, salads, and soups.

- Ask for substitutions. If you find a dish that you like, but it contains an ingredient that you can't eat, you can always ask the waiter or waitress to substitute something else. For example, you could ask for a salad without croutons, or a pasta dish without the sauce.

- Bring your own food. If you're really worried about not being able to find anything to eat, you can always bring your own food. This is a great option if you're going to a potluck or a party where you don't know what the food will be.

Communicating Your Dietary Needs to Others

Here are some tips for communicating your dietary needs to others:

- Be upfront about your condition. If you're going to be eating with someone who doesn't know about your CSID, it's important to let them know ahead of time. This will give them a chance to plan accordingly and make sure that there are foods that you can eat available.

- Be specific about your needs. Don't just say that you have a food allergy. Explain that you have CSID and that you can't eat sucrose or maltose. This will help people understand why you can't eat certain foods and what they need to do to accommodate your needs.

- Be patient. It may take some time for people to get used to your dietary needs. Be patient with them and don't get frustrated if they make mistakes. Just keep explaining your condition and what they need to do to help you.

- Don't be afraid to ask for help. If you're feeling overwhelmed or stressed, don't be afraid to ask for help from a friend, family member, or healthcare provider. They can help you navigate social situations and make sure that you're getting the support that you need.

COOKING AND MEAL PREPARATION FOR CSID:

Cooking and meal preparation are central to managing Congenital Sucrase-Isomaltase Deficiency (CSID) effectively. With careful planning and creative adaptations, you can enjoy a wide variety of delicious meals that are compatible with your dietary needs. By understanding CSID-compatible cooking techniques and exploring tailored recipes, you can maintain a well-rounded and satisfying diet while managing your symptoms.

CSID-Compatible Cooking Techniques:

CSID-friendly cooking techniques focus on breaking down complex carbohydrates and minimizing the intake of sucrose and isomaltose. Here are some cooking methods that align well with CSID dietary requirements:

- Grilling: Grilling meats, seafood, and vegetables is a great way to impart flavor without the need for added sugars or starches. Marinating with safe ingredients like olive oil, herbs, and spices can enhance taste.
- Roasting: Roasting vegetables, poultry, and fish can result in caramelization and depth of flavor without using high-sugar or starchy coatings.

- Steaming: Steaming is a gentle cooking method that retains nutrients and natural flavors. Steam vegetables and protein sources for a healthy and CSID-friendly meal.
- Baking: When baking, opt for recipes that use CSID-compatible flours and sweeteners. Almond flour, coconut flour, and mashed bananas can be alternatives in baking.
- Stir-Frying: Use minimal oil and stir-fry vegetables, lean proteins, and tofu to create flavorful dishes without relying on high-sugar sauces.
- Boiling: Boil vegetables, eggs, and proteins to create simple, easily digestible dishes. Be cautious with starches and added sugars in broths or sauces.

Delicious Recipes Tailored for CSID Patients:

Creating tasty meals that adhere to CSID dietary guidelines requires a bit of creativity. Here are a few recipe ideas that can be tailored to fit CSID needs

- **Zucchini Noodles with Pesto:** Replace traditional pasta with zucchini noodles and top them with a homemade pesto made from basil, pine nuts, olive oil, and Parmesan cheese (if tolerated).

- **Grilled Chicken and Veggie Skewers:** Thread pieces of marinated chicken, bell peppers, and zucchini onto skewers. Grill until cooked and serve with a side of quinoa or rice (in moderation) if allowed.

- **Baked Salmon with Lemon and Herbs:** Place a salmon fillet on a baking sheet, drizzle with lemon juice, sprinkle with fresh herbs like dill and parsley, and bake until flaky.

- **Stir-Fried Tofu and Broccoli:** Sauté tofu and broccoli in a minimal amount of oil with ginger, garlic, and low-sodium soy sauce for a flavorful stir-fry.

- **Egg and Spinach Breakfast Wrap:** Scramble eggs and sautéed spinach, then wrap the mixture in a large lettuce leaf for a nutritious breakfast or light meal.

- **Coconut Chia Pudding**: Mix chia seeds with coconut milk and a touch of vanilla extract. Let it sit overnight for a creamy and satisfying pudding.

- Fruit Parfait: Layer diced CSID-friendly fruits like berries, kiwi, and melon with dairy-free yogurt and a sprinkle of crushed nuts or seeds.

Remember, CSID-friendly recipes can be customized based on your specific tolerances and preferences. Experiment with different ingredients and cooking methods to find what works best for you while ensuring that your meals are both enjoyable and nutritious.

MONITORING PROGRESS AND SEEKING PROFESSIONAL GUIDANCE:

Living with a condition like Congenital Sucrase-Isomaltase Deficiency (CSID) requires a proactive approach to managing your health. Monitoring your progress and seeking professional guidance are essential components of effectively managing CSID and ensuring your well-being. By tracking your symptoms, noting improvements, and collaborating with healthcare providers and dietitians, you can make informed decisions and optimize your quality of life.

Tracking Symptoms and Improvements:

Regularly monitoring your symptoms and noting any improvements is crucial for understanding how your body responds to different foods and treatments. Here's how you can effectively track your progress:

- Symptom Journal: Keep a journal where you record your daily food intake, any symptoms you experience, their severity, and the timing of symptoms. This journal can help you identify patterns and potential triggers.

- Symptom Grading: Use a simple grading system to quantify the severity of symptoms. For example, use a scale from 1 to 10 to rate the intensity of symptoms like bloating, diarrhea, or stomach discomfort.

- Food Diary: Maintain a detailed food diary alongside your symptom journal. This will help you connect specific foods to symptom occurrences and identify safe options.

- Timeline of Changes: Create a timeline of dietary changes, medications, and treatments you've tried. This will provide valuable insights into what's working and what may need adjustments.

Collaborating with Healthcare Providers and Dietitians:

Medical professionals and dietitians are valuable allies in managing CSID effectively. Collaborating with them ensures that you receive expert guidance and personalized recommendations:

- Consulting a Gastroenterologist: A gastroenterologist specializing in digestive disorders like CSID can provide accurate diagnosis, treatment options, and regular check-ups. They can also perform relevant tests to monitor your progress.

- Registered Dietitian: A registered dietitian with expertise in CSID can help you create a tailored meal plan that ensures you're meeting your nutritional needs while avoiding trigger foods. They can also guide you through adapting recipes and making healthier choices.

- Regular Check-ups: Schedule regular appointments with your healthcare team to discuss your progress, share your symptom journal, and address any concerns. Adjustments to your treatment plan can be made based on their recommendations.

- Medication and Supplement Management: If your treatment plan involves medications or supplements, keep your healthcare provider informed about any changes in your symptoms or lifestyle. They can adjust dosages or recommend alternatives as needed.

- Emergency Plan: Work with your healthcare provider to create an emergency plan in case of severe symptoms or complications. Knowing when and how to seek medical attention can provide peace of mind.

In conclusion, monitoring your progress and seeking professional guidance are integral parts of managing CSID. By diligently tracking your symptoms, improvements, and dietary choices, you gain insights that empower you to make informed decisions. Collaborating with experienced healthcare providers and dietitians ensures that you receive personalized support and recommendations, leading to better management of your condition and an improved overall quality of life.

LIVING A FULL AND ENJOYABLE LIFE WITH CSID

Coping with Congenital Sucrase-Isomaltase Deficiency (CSID) can present unique challenges, but with the right strategies and mindset, individuals with CSID can still lead a vibrant and fulfilling life. By focusing on CSID-friendly social activities and nurturing emotional well-being with proper support, one can navigate the complexities of this condition while embracing a rich and enjoyable life.

CSID-Friendly Social Activities:

Engaging in social activities is an essential part of a well-rounded life, and having CSID doesn't mean missing out on these experiences. With a bit of planning and creativity, you can participate in various social gatherings while keeping your dietary restrictions in mind.

1. Potluck Parties with a Twist: Instead of dreading potluck events, consider hosting one with a theme that aligns with

your dietary needs. This way, you can ensure that there are plenty of CSID-friendly options available, while still enjoying the camaraderie of sharing a meal.

2. Cooking Workshops: Attend or organize cooking workshops that cater to individuals with dietary restrictions. Learning how to prepare delicious meals that suit your needs can empower you to enjoy food without worrying about triggering symptoms.

3. Outdoor Picnics and BBQs: Plan outdoor gatherings where you have more control over the menu. Grilled meats, vegetables, and fruit can be excellent choices for those with CSID.

4. Cultural Events: Explore cultural events and festivals that offer a variety of food options. Many cultures have dishes that naturally align with CSID dietary requirements, allowing you to savor new flavors without compromising your health.

Emotional Well-being and Support:

Managing CSID involves more than just dietary adjustments; emotional well-being plays a crucial role in leading a fulfilling life.

1. Open Communication: Talk openly with your friends, family, and close associates about your condition. Educate them about CSID, so they understand your limitations and can offer support.

2. Support Groups: Joining a CSID support group can provide you with a sense of belonging and a safe space to share experiences and advice. Connecting with others who understand your challenges can be immensely reassuring.

3. Mindfulness and Stress Management: Engage in mindfulness practices, meditation, or yoga to manage stress. Stress can exacerbate symptoms, so finding effective ways to reduce it can positively impact your well-being.

4. Professional Guidance: Consider seeking guidance from a mental health professional who specializes in chronic illnesses. They can help you navigate the emotional complexities that may arise due to living with CSID.

5. Celebrate Small Wins: Focus on your achievements and the progress you make in managing your CSID. Celebrate each step forward, whether it's finding a new CSID-friendly recipe or successfully navigating a social event.

In conclusion, living a full and enjoyable life with CSID is absolutely achievable. By embracing CSID-friendly social activities and prioritizing your emotional well-being, you can create a fulfilling lifestyle that not only accommodates your dietary needs but also nurtures your happiness and sense of connection with others. Remember, CSID is just one aspect of your life, and with the right approach, you can continue to thrive and savor every moment.

FREQUENTLY ASKED QUESTIONS ABOUT CSID

What is CSID?

CSID is a rare genetic disorder that affects the body's ability to digest sucrose and starch. Sucrase and isomaltase are enzymes that are needed to break down these sugars in the small intestine. When someone has CSID, they do not have enough of these enzymes, which can lead to symptoms such as diarrhea, bloating, gas, and abdominal pain after eating foods that contain sucrose or starch.

How is CSID diagnosed?

CSID is typically diagnosed in infants or young children who experience symptoms after eating sugary or starchy foods. A doctor can diagnose CSID with a blood test or a breath test. The blood test measures the levels of sucrase and isomaltase in the blood. The breath test measures the amount of hydrogen in the breath after a person drinks a solution that contains sucrose. If the levels of sucrase and isomaltase are low, or if the amount of hydrogen in the breath is high, this can be a sign of CSID.

How is CSID treated?

There is no cure for CSID, but it can be managed with diet and medication. The goal of treatment is to avoid or limit foods that contain sucrose and starch. Some people with CSID may be able to tolerate small amounts of these foods, but others may need to strictly avoid them. There is also a medication called Sucraid® that can help to improve digestion of sucrose in people with CSID.

What are the common symptoms of CSID?

The most common symptoms of CSID are diarrhea, bloating, gas, and abdominal pain after eating foods that contain sucrose or starch. Other symptoms can include nausea, vomiting, and weight loss. Symptoms can be mild or severe, and they can vary from person to person.

What are the complications of CSID?

If CSID is not managed properly, it can lead to dehydration, malnutrition, and weight loss. In severe cases, CSID can lead to kidney damage.

Can CSID be prevented?

There is no way to prevent CSID, as it is a genetic disorder. However, early diagnosis and treatment can help to prevent complications.

What is the life expectancy for people with CSID?

People with CSID can have a normal life expectancy if they are diagnosed and treated early. With proper management, people with CSID can live healthy and active lives.

What are the challenges of living with CSID?

One of the biggest challenges of living with CSID is managing the diet. People with CSID need to be very careful about what they eat, as even small amounts of sucrose and starch can cause symptoms. This can be difficult, especially when eating out or at social events. Another challenge of living with CSID is the social stigma that can be associated with the disorder. People with CSID may be accused of being picky eaters or of having an eating disorder. It is important to remember that CSID is a real medical condition, and that people with CSID are not to blame for their symptoms.

What are the resources available for people with CSID?

There are a number of resources available for people with CSID and their families. The National Organization for Rare Disorders (NORD) has a website with information about CSID, as well as a support group for people with the disorder. There are also a number of private organizations that provide support and resources for people with CSID.

How do I know if I have CSID?

If you are experiencing symptoms of CSID, such as diarrhea, bloating, gas, and abdominal pain after eating sugary or starchy foods, it is important to see a doctor for diagnosis. There is no one-size-fits-all test for CSID, but your doctor may order a blood test or a breath test to help make a diagnosis.

Conclusion

In conclusion, I hope that the meal plans, recipes, and information provided in this book have been valuable in helping you navigate life with Congenital Sucrase-Isomaltase Deficiency (CSID). Your journey towards managing your condition while still enjoying a fulfilling and delicious diet is both inspiring and important. If you have found this book to be beneficial in any way, I encourage you to take a moment to share your experience with others.

Your feedback is invaluable in spreading awareness and knowledge about CSID-friendly living. By rating and reviewing this book, you can contribute to a growing community of individuals who are seeking practical solutions and support for managing their CSID. Your words have the power to inspire others to embark on their own path towards wellness and joy.

Thank you for being a part of this journey. Together, we can create a supportive and informed network that empowers individuals with CSID to live their lives to the fullest while embracing health, happiness, and a love for good food.